# HERBAL TINCTURE FOR ENHANCED WELLNESS

## Organic Extract for Vitality & Health from nature - 5-in-1 Support

### David D. Lucero

# CONTENTS

# PREFACE

Welcome to "Herbal Tincture for Wellness." This book is a comprehensive exploration of the world of herbal tinctures—a time-honored form of herbal medicine aimed at promoting well-being and vitality.

Herbal tinctures have been used for centuries as a natural approach to support health and address various ailments. By extracting the medicinal properties of herbs into a concentrated liquid form, tinctures offer a convenient and potent way to harness the healing potential of nature.

Within these pages, you'll embark on a journey through the fundamentals of herbal tinctures: from understanding the extraction process and selecting herbs to creating your own tinctures tailored to specific wellness goals. This book endeavors to provide insights into the diverse range of herbs used in tincture-making, their potential health benefits, and guidelines for their safe and effective use.

It's important to note that while herbal tinctures can offer holistic support for well-being, individual responses and health conditions vary. Consultation with a qualified healthcare professional is advised before incorporating herbal tinctures into your wellness regimen, especially if you have pre-existing health concerns or are taking medications.

I extend my gratitude to the herbalists, practitioners, and enthusiasts whose knowledge and dedication have contributed to the preservation and advancement of herbal medicine. Furthermore, I commend the readers who seek to explore the natural remedies offered by herbal tinctures on their path toward holistic wellness.

May this book serve as a trusted guide in your quest to embrace the healing powers of herbal tinctures and nurture a balanced and vibrant life.

Warm regards.

# INTRODUCTION



Herbal tinctures are concentrated liquid extracts derived from herbs and plants, typically utilizing a combination of alcohol and water as a solvent. This extraction method preserves and concentrates the active compounds present in the plant material, making it a potent and effective form of herbal medicine. The term "tincture" itself refers to the alcohol-based extraction process, distinguishing it from other herbal preparations like infusions or decoctions.

**Key Characteristics of Herbal Tinctures:**

- **Concentration:** Herbal tinctures are highly concentrated, containing a higher proportion of active ingredients compared to other forms of herbal remedies.

- **Solvents:** The most common solvent used is alcohol, which effectively extracts both water-soluble and alcohol-soluble components from the plant material.

- **Long Shelf Life:** Due to the alcohol content, tinctures have a longer shelf life compared to some other herbal preparations.

## Advantages of Herbal Tinctures:

1. **Efficiency:** Tinctures offer a more efficient extraction of medicinal compounds, requiring smaller doses for therapeutic effects.

2. **Ease of Administration:** Tinctures are easy to administer, with most people finding the liquid form more palatable than capsules or tablets.

3. **Quick Absorption:** The liquid form allows for faster absorption into the bloodstream, facilitating a rapid onset of therapeutic effects.

## How Herbal Tinctures Are Made:

1. **Harvesting:** The process begins with the careful harvesting of plant material, ensuring it is at its peak in terms of medicinal potency.

2. **Chopping or Grinding:** The plant material is then chopped or ground to increase the surface area for extraction.

3. **Maceration:** The chopped or ground material is soaked in a mixture of alcohol and water, allowing the solvent to extract the active compounds.

4. **Straining:** After a designated maceration period, the liquid is strained to remove plant residues, leaving behind a concentrated herbal extract.

5. **Bottling:** The final tincture is then bottled, often in dark glass containers to protect it from light, and labeled with dosage instructions.

## Overview of Tincture Extraction Process

The tincture extraction process is a meticulous and artful method of transforming botanicals into potent remedies. Understanding the key steps involved sheds light on the efficacy and quality of the final product.

## Alcohol as a Solvent:

- **Preservation:** Alcohol serves as an excellent preservative, preventing the growth of bacteria and fungi in the tincture.

- **Extraction Medium:** Alcohol is a versatile solvent, effectively extracting both water-soluble and fat-soluble compounds from the plant material.

## Ratio of Alcohol to Water:

- **Varied Ratios:** Different herbs require different ratios of alcohol to water. Some herbs benefit from a higher alcohol content, while others are best extracted with a higher water content.

## Maceration Duration:

- **Time Sensitivity:** The duration of maceration significantly impacts the final product. Too short a maceration may result in an under-extracted tincture, while too long may lead to over-extraction and a bitter taste.

## Quality of Ingredients:

- **Selecting Fresh Herbs:** The quality of the tincture heavily relies on the freshness and quality of the herbs used. Fresh, high-quality herbs yield more potent extracts.

## Filtering and Bottling:

- **Precision in Filtration:** Proper filtration ensures the removal of plant material, preventing sedimentation in the final tincture.

- **Dark Glass Bottles:** The use of dark glass bottles

protects the tincture from light, which can degrade its potency.

# Historical Significance In Traditional Medicine

The use of herbal tinctures has a rich history deeply intertwined with traditional medicine practices across cultures. This historical significance provides insight into the enduring efficacy and cultural value of tinctures.

**Ancient Roots:**

- **Ancient Civilizations:** Various ancient civilizations, including the Egyptians, Greeks, and Chinese, incorporated herbal tinctures into their medicinal practices.

- **Alchemical Traditions:** The alchemical traditions of the Middle Ages also contributed to the development of tinctures, viewing them as potent elixirs with transformative properties.

**Traditional Western Herbalism:**

- **Influence of Eclecticism:** In the 19th and early 20th centuries, eclectic herbalism in the West embraced tinctures as a versatile and effective form of herbal medicine.

- **Continued Use:** Traditional Western herbalism continues to rely on tinctures for their therapeutic benefits.

**Ayurveda and Traditional Chinese Medicine:**

- **Ayurvedic Tinctures:** In Ayurveda, the traditional medicine of India, tinctures are used as part of holistic healing practices.

- **Chinese Medicinal Wines:** Traditional Chinese

Medicine incorporates medicinal wines, a form of herbal tincture, for both internal and external applications.

**Shamanic and Indigenous Practices:**

- **Connection with Nature:** Indigenous cultures globally have integrated herbal tinctures into shamanic and folk healing practices, emphasizing a deep connection with nature.

- **Cultural Preservation:** The use of tinctures in indigenous medicine highlights the preservation of cultural knowledge and the importance of sustainable herbal practices.

# BENEFITS OF HERBAL TINCTURES

*Health and Wellness*

In the fast-paced world we inhabit, prioritizing health and wellness is essential for leading a fulfilling life. Health and wellness encompass a holistic approach to physical, mental, and emotional well-being. It involves making conscious choices to maintain a balanced and harmonious existence. Aiming for optimal health involves adopting healthy lifestyle habits, including regular exercise, a nutritious diet, and adequate sleep.

**1. Regular Exercise:** Regular physical activity is the cornerstone of good health. Engaging in exercise not only improves cardiovascular health but also boosts mood and reduces the risk of chronic diseases. From brisk walks to intense workouts, finding an activity that suits your preferences can make a significant difference in your overall well-being.

**2. Nutritious Diet:** A well-balanced diet is vital for supplying the body with the necessary nutrients for optimal functioning. Incorporating a variety of fruits, vegetables, whole grains, and lean proteins can provide the body with the fuel it needs. Moreover, staying hydrated is crucial for maintaining bodily functions and supporting overall health.

**3. Adequate Sleep:** Quality sleep is often underestimated but plays a pivotal role in health and wellness. Establishing a consistent sleep routine helps the body and mind recharge, promoting cognitive function, emotional well-being, and immune system support.

## Immune System Support

The immune system is the body's defense mechanism against harmful invaders, such as bacteria, viruses, and other pathogens. Strengthening the immune system is crucial for maintaining good health and preventing illness.

**1. Balanced Nutrition:** A well-nourished body is better equipped to fend off infections and diseases. Essential nutrients like vitamins C and D, zinc, and antioxidants contribute to a robust immune system. These nutrients can be obtained from a diverse and balanced diet that includes fruits, vegetables, whole grains, and lean proteins.

**2. Regular Exercise:** Exercise not only benefits physical health but also enhances immune function. Moderate-intensity exercise has been shown to promote healthy immune responses. It's important to strike a balance, as excessive exercise may have the opposite effect on immune function.

**3. Sufficient Sleep:** Sleep is when the body undergoes crucial repair and regeneration processes, including the strengthening of the immune system. Chronic sleep deprivation can impair immune function, making it essential to prioritize restful and adequate sleep.

## Stress Relief And Mental Well-Being

In our modern, fast-paced lives, stress has become a prevalent concern. Managing stress and prioritizing mental well-being are integral components of a healthy lifestyle.

**1. Mindfulness Practices:** Mindfulness techniques, such as meditation and deep breathing exercises, can help reduce stress and promote mental clarity. Incorporating these practices into daily routines fosters a sense of calm and balance.

**2. Adequate Rest:** Ensuring sufficient downtime is crucial for mental well-being. It's essential to strike a balance between work and rest, allowing the mind to relax and recharge. Establishing healthy sleep patterns contributes significantly to stress relief.

**3. Social Connections:** Maintaining strong social connections is a powerful stress-reliever. Engaging with friends and family provides emotional support and a sense of belonging, reducing feelings of isolation and stress.

## Natural Healing Properties

Nature has long been a source of healing, providing remedies for various ailments. Exploring natural healing properties involves tapping into the therapeutic benefits of plants, herbs, and other natural elements.

**1. Herbal Remedies:** Herbs have been used for centuries for their medicinal properties. From soothing chamomile tea to immune-boosting echinacea, herbal remedies offer a natural alternative for various health concerns.

**2. Aromatherapy:** Aromatherapy harnesses the power of scents to influence mood and well-being. Essential oils derived from plants have diverse therapeutic effects, from promoting relaxation to boosting energy levels.

**3. Nature Therapy:** Spending time in nature, known as ecotherapy or nature therapy, has been linked to reduced stress levels and improved mental health. Whether it's a walk in the woods or simply enjoying a garden, connecting with nature can have profound healing effects.

## Anti-Inflammatory Effects

Inflammation is a natural response to injury or infection, but chronic inflammation can contribute to various health problems. Understanding and incorporating anti-inflammatory practices into our lives is key to preventing and managing inflammation.

**1. Omega-3 Fatty Acids:** Found in fatty fish, flaxseeds, and walnuts, omega-3 fatty acids possess anti-inflammatory properties. Including these foods in your diet can help reduce inflammation and support overall health.

**2. Turmeric and Curcumin:** Turmeric, a spice commonly used in Indian cuisine, contains curcumin, a potent anti-inflammatory compound. Incorporating turmeric into your diet or taking curcumin supplements may help manage inflammation.

**3. Regular Exercise:** Exercise not only supports overall

health but also has anti-inflammatory effects. Engaging in regular physical activity helps regulate the body's inflammatory responses and reduces the risk of chronic inflammation.

## Antioxidant Benefits

Antioxidants play a crucial role in protecting the body from oxidative stress, which can contribute to aging and various diseases. Incorporating antioxidant-rich foods into your diet is a proactive way to support overall health.

**1. Berries:** Berries, such as blueberries, strawberries, and raspberries, are rich in antioxidants. These compounds help neutralize free radicals, reducing oxidative stress and supporting cellular health.

**2. Dark Chocolate:** Dark chocolate contains flavonoids, which have antioxidant properties. Consuming moderate amounts of high-quality dark chocolate can contribute to antioxidant benefits while satisfying sweet cravings.

**3. Colorful Vegetables:** Vegetables with vibrant colors, such as spinach, kale, and bell peppers, are rich in antioxidants like vitamins A, C, and E. Including a variety of colorful vegetables in your diet provides a broad spectrum of antioxidant benefits.

# POPULAR HERBS FOR TINCTURE MAKING

*Echinacea*

Echinacea, a vibrant and resilient flower, has long been celebrated for its potential health benefits. Renowned for its immune-boosting properties, Echinacea is a popular choice for those seeking natural remedies to support their well-being. The plant is native to North America and has been used by indigenous peoples for centuries. Its medicinal qualities are derived from the roots, leaves, and flowers. Let's delve into the key components that contribute to Echinacea's remarkable immune-boosting properties:

1. **Alkamides:** Echinacea contains alkamides, which are compounds that play a crucial role in modulating the immune system. These alkamides interact with various receptors in the body, enhancing the overall immune response.

2. **Polyphenols:** Rich in polyphenols, Echinacea exhibits potent antioxidant properties. These compounds help neutralize free radicals, reducing oxidative stress and supporting the immune system's ability to function optimally.

3. **Polysaccharides:** Echinacea's polysaccharides contribute to its immune-boosting effects. These complex carbohydrates stimulate the activity of white blood cells, enhancing the body's defense mechanisms.

4. **Caffeic Acid Derivatives:** Another key component, caffeic acid derivatives, exhibits anti-inflammatory effects. This contributes to Echinacea's ability to mitigate inflammation, allowing the immune system to focus on combating potential threats.

The immune-boosting properties of Echinacea make it a popular choice during cold and flu seasons. Its versatility, available in various forms such as capsules, tinctures, and teas, allows individuals to incorporate it into their wellness routines in a way that suits their preferences.

## Immune-Boosting Properties

Understanding the intricacies of immune-boosting properties is vital in maintaining overall health. A robust immune system serves as the body's defense against pathogens, preventing infections and promoting well-being. **Let's explore the key elements that contribute to enhancing the immune system:**

1. **Vitamins and Minerals:** Adequate intake of essential vitamins and minerals is paramount for immune function. Vitamin C, vitamin D, zinc, and selenium are among the nutrients crucial for supporting the immune system.

2. **Antioxidants:** Antioxidants play a pivotal role in neutralizing free radicals that can compromise immune function. Incorporating a variety of fruits, vegetables, and herbs rich in antioxidants, such as Echinacea, can bolster the body's defenses.

3. **Probiotics:** A healthy gut is closely linked to a strong immune system. Probiotics, often referred to as "good" bacteria, promote gut health and contribute to the overall balance of the immune system.

4. **Regular Exercise:** Physical activity has been shown to have a positive impact on the immune system. Moderate, consistent exercise can enhance immune function and contribute to overall well-being.

Understanding these components empowers individuals to make informed choices in supporting their immune health. By adopting a holistic approach that includes a balanced diet, regular exercise, and incorporating immune-boosting herbs like Echinacea, individuals can fortify their bodies against external threats.

## Proper Extraction Techniques

The efficacy of herbal remedies, such as Echinacea, relies significantly on the extraction techniques employed. Proper extraction ensures that the beneficial compounds present in the plant are retained in the final product. **Let's explore the key extraction techniques that maximize the potency of herbal remedies:**

1. **Cold Infusion:** This gentle method involves soaking the herbs in cold water for an extended period. While it takes more time, cold infusion helps preserve delicate compounds that might be damaged by heat, ensuring a more comprehensive extraction.

2. **Tinctures:** Tinctures involve steeping herbs in a mixture of alcohol and water. This method is efficient in extracting both water-soluble and alcohol-soluble compounds, resulting in a concentrated and easily absorbed form of the herb.

3. **Decoction:** Suitable for tougher plant materials like roots and bark, decoction involves simmering the herbs in water. This method is effective in extracting the more robust, less water-soluble compounds.

4. **Steam Distillation:** Commonly used for essential oils, steam distillation involves passing steam through the plant material, causing the essential oils to evaporate. The condensed vapor contains the concentrated plant compounds.

Choosing the right extraction method depends on the properties of the herb and the desired outcome. For Echinacea, a combination of extraction techniques may be employed to capture the diverse range of beneficial compounds it contains.

# Lavender

Lavender, with its captivating fragrance and soothing properties, transcends its role as a garden favorite. This versatile herb has been cherished for centuries for its diverse applications, ranging from aromatherapy to culinary delights. **Let's explore the multifaceted aspects of lavender and how it contributes to stress reduction and relaxation:**

1. **Aromatherapy:** The aroma of lavender is known to have calming effects on the nervous system. Inhaling lavender essential oil can reduce stress and anxiety, promoting a sense of relaxation.

2. **Sedative Properties:** Lavender contains compounds with mild sedative effects. These compounds interact with neurotransmitters, such as GABA, promoting a calming response in the brain.

3. **Topical Applications:** Lavender oil can be applied topically to promote relaxation. Diluted lavender oil may be used in massages or added to bathwater, providing a sensory experience that eases tension and promotes overall well-being.

4. **Sleep Aid:** Lavender is renowned for its sleep-inducing properties. Incorporating lavender sachets in the bedroom or using lavender-infused products can contribute to a restful night's sleep.

Lavender's ability to induce relaxation makes it a valuable

tool in managing stress in our fast-paced lives. Whether in the form of essential oils, teas, or as part of self-care rituals, lavender continues to be a cherished ally in promoting tranquility.

## Stress Reduction And Relaxation

In the hustle and bustle of modern life, stress reduction and relaxation are paramount for maintaining mental and physical well-being. **Let's explore effective strategies for managing stress and fostering a sense of relaxation:**

1. **Mindfulness and Meditation:** Practices like mindfulness and meditation can help calm the mind and reduce stress. These techniques involve focusing on the present moment, promoting a sense of tranquility.

2. **Physical Activity:** Regular exercise is a powerful stress buster. Engaging in physical activity releases endorphins, the body's natural mood lifters, and helps alleviate tension.

3. **Quality Sleep:** Prioritizing a good night's sleep is crucial for stress management. Establishing a consistent sleep routine and creating a comfortable sleep environment contribute to overall well-being.

4. **Social Connections:** Building and maintaining positive social connections provide emotional support, reducing feelings of isolation and stress. Spending time with loved ones fosters a sense of belonging.

## Crafting Lavender Tinctures

Crafting lavender tinctures allows individuals to harness the therapeutic properties of this aromatic herb. Tinctures, concentrated herbal extracts, are a versatile way to incorporate lavender into daily wellness routines. **Let's explore the steps involved in crafting lavender tinctures and how to make the most of this herbal preparation:**

1. **Harvesting Lavender:** Choose fresh lavender flowers for optimal potency. Harvest when the flowers are in full bloom, typically in the morning when the essential oil content is highest.

2. **Preparing the Tincture Base:** Use high-proof alcohol, such as vodka or brandy, as the solvent for extracting lavender's beneficial compounds. The alcohol acts as a preservative and efficiently extracts both water-soluble and alcohol-soluble constituents.

3. **Ratio and Measurement:** Maintain a proper ratio of lavender to alcohol. A common ratio is one part dried lavender flowers to two parts alcohol. Use a glass jar with a tight-fitting lid for the tincture-making process.

4. **Extraction Time:** Allow the lavender and alcohol mixture to steep for several weeks, shaking the jar regularly. This prolonged extraction period ensures a potent tincture.

5. **Straining and Bottling:** After the extraction period, strain the tincture to remove plant material. Transfer the liquid into dark glass bottles to protect the tincture from light, preserving its potency.

Crafted lavender tinctures can be used in various ways, from adding a few drops to beverages or using them topically for a calming massage. This DIY approach empowers individuals to create a personalized lavender-infused experience tailored to their preferences and wellness goals.

# DIY HERBAL TINCTURE RECIPES

*Step-by-Step Guide to*
*Tincture Preparation*

Creating herbal tinctures at home is a rewarding and therapeutic endeavor. Follow this step-by-step guide to master the art of tincture preparation.

**1. Choose Your Herbs:** Before embarking on your tincture-making journey, carefully select the herbs you want to use. The quality and freshness of the herbs significantly impact the potency of the tincture. Whether it's for medicinal or culinary purposes, research the properties of each herb to ensure they align with your goals.

**2. Gather Supplies:** Assemble all the necessary materials. You'll need high-proof alcohol (like vodka or Everclear), glass jars with tight-fitting lids, and, of course, your chosen herbs. Ensure that the jars are clean and sterile to prevent contamination.

**3. Measure and Chop:** Precise measurements are crucial for a potent tincture. Use a scale to measure the herbs accurately. Once measured, chop or grind the herbs. This increases the surface area, allowing the alcohol to extract the beneficial compounds more efficiently.

**4. Combine Herbs and Alcohol:** Place the chopped herbs in the glass jar, and cover them with the chosen alcohol. The ratio of herbs to alcohol varies based on the herb's potency, but a common ratio is one part herbs to two parts alcohol. Seal the jar tightly.

**5. Shake and Store:** Shake the jar vigorously to ensure the herbs are thoroughly coated with alcohol. Store the jar in a cool, dark place, like a pantry or cupboard, for at least two to six weeks. Remember to shake the jar periodically to promote optimal extraction.

**6. Strain and Bottle:** After the steeping period, strain the mixture using cheesecloth or a fine mesh sieve to remove plant material. Squeeze the herbs to extract every bit of liquid. Funnel the resulting tincture into dark glass bottles, which protect the contents from light, preserving their medicinal properties.

**7. Label and Date:** Accurate labeling is essential. Clearly mark the bottle with the name of the herb, the type of alcohol used, and the date of preparation. This ensures you keep track of expiration dates and the tincture's effectiveness over time.

## Choosing The Right Herbs

Selecting the right herbs for your tincture is a crucial step that requires careful consideration. Here are some key points to guide your herb selection process.

**1. Know Your Purpose:** Define the purpose of your tincture. Are you creating it for medicinal reasons, like immune support or stress relief? Alternatively, is it for culinary use, adding unique flavors to your dishes? Knowing your objective helps narrow down the herb choices.

**2. Research Herbal Properties:** Thoroughly research the properties of each herb under consideration. Some herbs are renowned for their calming effects, while others are prized for their immune-boosting properties. Understanding these qualities ensures your tincture aligns with your desired outcomes.

**3. Consider Flavor Profiles:** If you're crafting a culinary tincture, consider the flavor profiles of different herbs. Some herbs, like basil or thyme, can enhance savory dishes, while others, like mint or lavender, complement sweet treats. Experiment with combinations to find the perfect blend.

**4. Seasonal and Local:** Whenever possible, choose herbs that are in season and locally sourced. Fresh, seasonal herbs tend to be more potent and flavorful. Supporting local farmers also contributes to sustainability and promotes a connection to your community.

**5. Check Compatibility:** Some herbs work synergistically, enhancing each other's effects, while others may have conflicting properties. Before combining herbs, ensure they are compatible and won't negate each other's benefits.

## Alcohol Vs. Vinegar Extraction Methods

The choice between alcohol and vinegar as extraction

methods for herbal tinctures depends on various factors, including the type of herbs and intended use.

## 1. Alcohol Extraction:

- **Pros:**
  - Efficient extraction of medicinal compounds.
  - Longer shelf life.
  - Versatility in creating tinctures for various purposes.

- **Cons:**
  - High-proof alcohol can be expensive.
  - Not suitable for individuals avoiding alcohol consumption.
  - Some herbs may lose flavor nuances.

Alcohol extraction is the most common method due to its effectiveness in extracting a broad spectrum of compounds. It is particularly suitable for tinctures intended for medicinal use, as alcohol efficiently captures the active constituents of the herbs.

## 2. Vinegar Extraction:

- **Pros:**
  - Budget-friendly alternative to alcohol.
  - Suitable for individuals avoiding alcohol.
  - Preserves the herb's flavor nuances.

- **Cons:**
  - Shorter shelf life compared to alcohol-based tinctures.
  - May not extract certain compounds as effectively.

Vinegar extraction is an excellent option for those who prefer an alcohol-free tincture. It's budget-friendly and preserves the flavors of the herbs, making it a popular choice for culinary applications.

## Sample Recipes

### Immune-Boosting Echinacea Blend

**Ingredients:**

- 1 part dried echinacea
- 2 parts high-proof alcohol (vodka or Everclear)

**Instructions:**

1. Weigh the dried echinacea and chop it finely.
2. Place the echinacea in a glass jar and cover it with the alcohol.
3. Seal the jar tightly and shake it thoroughly.
4. Store in a cool, dark place for 4-6 weeks, shaking periodically.
5. Strain the tincture and transfer it to a dark glass bottle.
6. Label with the herb name, alcohol type, and preparation date.

### Calming Lavender Infusion

**Ingredients:**

- 1 part dried lavender
- 2 parts apple cider vinegar

**Instructions:**

1. Weigh the dried lavender and chop it finely.

2. Place the lavender in a glass jar and cover it with the apple cider vinegar.

3. Seal the jar tightly and shake it thoroughly.

4. Store in a cool, dark place for 2-4 weeks, shaking periodically.

5. Strain the tincture and transfer it to a dark glass bottle.

6. Label with the herb name, vinegar type, and preparation date.

These sample recipes provide a starting point for creating tinctures tailored to your needs, whether for immune support or a calming culinary experience. Experimenting with different herbs and ratios allows you to discover unique blends that resonate with your preferences and health goals.

# UNDERSTANDING DOSAGES AND USAGE

## Dos and Don'ts of Herbal Tincture Consumption

Herbal tinctures have been embraced for centuries as a natural remedy for various ailments. However, navigating the dos and don'ts of their consumption is crucial for ensuring their effectiveness and safety.

## Dos

### 1. Research Thoroughly Before Use

Before incorporating any herbal tincture into your routine, conduct comprehensive research. Understand the properties, benefits, and potential side effects of the specific herb. This knowledge empowers you to make informed decisions about your health.

## 2. Purchase from Reputable Sources

The quality of herbal tinctures varies, and sourcing them from reputable suppliers is essential. Choose products from trusted brands or herbalists who prioritize quality and adhere to ethical standards in cultivation and production.

## 3. Start with Small Dosages

Introduce herbal tinctures gradually. Start with a small dosage to assess your body's reaction. Monitoring how your body responds allows you to adjust the dosage accordingly, preventing adverse effects.

## 4. Be Consistent with Dosage

Consistency is key when consuming herbal tinctures. Establish a routine that suits your lifestyle, ensuring you take the recommended dosage regularly. Regularity enhances the tincture's efficacy over time.

## 5. Mix with Water or Juice

Many herbal tinctures have potent flavors that may not be palatable on their own. To make consumption more pleasant, mix the recommended dosage with water or juice. This not only improves taste but also aids absorption.

## 6. Monitor Your Body's Response

Pay close attention to how your body responds to herbal tinctures. Look for positive effects, such as improved mood or reduced symptoms. Equally, be vigilant for any negative reactions, and consult a healthcare professional if needed.

# Don'ts

## 1. Exceed Recommended Dosages

More is not always better when it comes to herbal tinctures. Exceeding recommended dosages can lead to adverse effects and toxicity. Stick to the guidelines provided by healthcare professionals or product labels.

## 2. Self-Diagnose Serious Conditions

While herbal tinctures can complement conventional medicine, they should not be used to self-diagnose or treat serious medical conditions. Consult with a healthcare professional for a proper diagnosis and treatment plan.

## 3. Disregard Potential Interactions

Herbal tinctures may interact with medications or exacerbate existing health conditions. Always disclose your herbal tincture use to your healthcare provider to ensure compatibility with other treatments.

## 4. Assume One Size Fits All

Each individual's body responds differently to herbal tinctures. Avoid assuming that a dosage suitable for someone else will work for you. Tailor your consumption based on your unique health needs and responses.

## 5. Ignore Quality Concerns

Poor-quality herbal tinctures may contain contaminants or lack the desired medicinal properties. Ignoring quality concerns can compromise your health. Invest in products from trustworthy sources to guarantee the purity and efficacy of the tincture.

## 6. Rely Solely on Herbal Remedies for Chronic Conditions

While herbal tinctures can be beneficial, they should not replace conventional medical treatments for chronic or severe conditions. Consult with healthcare professionals to integrate herbal remedies into a comprehensive treatment plan.

# Consultation With Healthcare Professionals

Embarking on a journey of herbal tincture consumption requires more than just personal research. Consulting with healthcare professionals adds an extra layer of safety and ensures that your health goals align with your overall well-being.

# Dos

## 1. Inform Your Healthcare Provider

Always inform your healthcare provider about your intention to incorporate herbal tinctures into your health regimen. This transparency enables them to provide guidance, considering potential interactions with existing medications or health conditions.

## 2. Seek Professional Advice on Herb Selection

Healthcare professionals can offer valuable insights into

the selection of herbs based on your specific health needs. Their expertise helps tailor your herbal regimen to address your unique symptoms or conditions effectively.

### 3. Regular Health Check-ups

Schedule regular check-ups with your healthcare provider to monitor your overall health. These check-ups can identify any changes or improvements in your condition, allowing for adjustments to your herbal tincture consumption if necessary.

### 4. Collaborate for Holistic Healthcare

Collaborate with healthcare professionals to create a holistic healthcare plan. Integrating herbal tinctures into this plan ensures that they complement, rather than contradict, other aspects of your health management.

## Don'ts

### 1. Neglect Professional Advice

While personal research is valuable, it should not replace the advice of healthcare professionals. Neglecting their guidance may lead to unintended consequences, especially if there are underlying health issues.

### 2. Assume All Healthcare Providers Are Familiar with Herbal Remedies

Not all healthcare providers may be well-versed in herbal remedies. If your primary healthcare provider lacks expertise in this area, consider seeking advice from specialists or herbalists who can provide tailored guidance.

### 3. Discontinue Conventional Medications Without Approval

Herbal tinctures are not always a substitute for conventional medications. Do not discontinue prescribed medications without the approval of your healthcare provider, as this can negatively impact your health.

## 4. Overlook Changes in Health Status

Any changes in your health status, whether positive or negative, should be communicated to your healthcare provider. Overlooking these changes may result in an inaccurate assessment of the effectiveness of herbal tinctures.

## 5. Assume Herbal Remedies Are Risk-Free

While herbal remedies are generally considered safe, they are not entirely risk-free. Some individuals may experience allergies or adverse reactions. Reporting such incidents promptly to healthcare professionals is crucial for appropriate management.

## 6. Delay Seeking Professional Help for Adverse Reactions

If you experience adverse reactions to herbal tinctures, do not delay seeking professional help. Healthcare providers can guide you through managing side effects or determining whether the herbal remedy is suitable for you.

# Tailoring Dosages To Individual Needs

One size does not fit all when it comes to herbal tincture consumption. Tailoring dosages to individual needs is a crucial aspect that maximizes benefits while minimizing potential risks.

# Dos

## 1. Understand Personal Health Goals

Clearly define your health goals before incorporating herbal tinctures. Whether it's managing stress, improving sleep, or addressing specific symptoms, understanding your objectives helps tailor the dosage to meet your individual needs.

## 2. Start with Low Dosages

Initiate your herbal tincture journey with lower dosages. This cautious approach allows you to assess your body's response and make gradual adjustments. Starting low and increasing incrementally minimizes the risk of adverse effects.

## 3. Keep a Dosage Journal

Maintain a dosage journal to track your consumption and its effects. Note any changes in symptoms, mood, or overall well-being. This journal becomes a valuable tool for adjusting dosages based on your body's responses over time.

## 4. Consider Body Weight and Metabolism

Individual factors such as body weight and metabolism play a role in how herbal tinctures are absorbed and utilized. Adjust dosages accordingly, with guidance from healthcare professionals, to ensure optimal efficacy for your unique physiology.

# Don'ts

## 1. Follow Generic Dosage Recommendations Blindly

Generic dosage recommendations may not account for individual variations. Blindly following these recommendations can result in either suboptimal effects or, in some cases, adverse reactions. Always customize dosages based on individual needs.

## 2. Ignore Changes in Symptoms

If your symptoms change or evolve, do not ignore these shifts. They may indicate the need for dosage adjustments or a reassessment of the herbal tincture's suitability for your current health status.

## 3. Assume Higher Dosages Are Always Better

The belief that higher dosages equate to better results is a misconception. Excessive dosages can overwhelm the body and lead to adverse effects. Always prioritize the effectiveness of the herbal tincture over the quantity consumed.

## 4. Neglect Professional Guidance

Tailoring dosages requires a nuanced understanding of herbal properties and individual health factors. Neglecting professional guidance can result in suboptimal outcomes or unintended consequences for your health.

## 5. Disregard Changes in Lifestyle

Changes in lifestyle, such as alterations in diet or exercise, can influence how herbal tinctures interact with your body. Keep healthcare professionals informed about such changes to ensure dosages remain aligned with your evolving health needs.

## 6. Delay Adjustments for Persistent Issues

If you encounter persistent issues or lack of improvement,

do not delay in adjusting dosages. Consult with healthcare professionals promptly to address concerns and explore alternative approaches to optimize your herbal tincture experience.

# SAFETY AND STORAGE

## *Proper Storage Techniques*

**P**roper storage techniques are paramount when it comes to maintaining the quality and safety of various products, ranging from food items to pharmaceuticals. The significance of proper storage extends beyond just keeping things organized; it directly influences the longevity and efficacy of the stored items.

**Temperature Control:** One of the key factors in proper storage is temperature control. Different products have different temperature requirements for optimal preservation. For instance, perishable food items generally require refrigeration to slow down bacterial growth, while certain chemicals may need to be stored at specific temperatures to prevent degradation.

**Humidity Management:** Humidity plays a critical role in the storage of many items. Excessive moisture can lead to mold growth, spoilage of food, and degradation of various materials. On the other hand, extremely dry conditions can result in the drying out and deterioration of certain products. Maintaining the right balance of humidity is crucial for preserving the integrity of stored items.

**Proper Ventilation:** Adequate ventilation is often overlooked but is crucial in preventing the buildup of odors, gases, or moisture that can compromise the quality of stored goods. Proper airflow helps maintain a consistent environment, preventing the formation of pockets of stagnant air that may foster the growth of bacteria or the development of undesirable odors.

**Light Exposure:** Some products are sensitive to light exposure, which can lead to chemical reactions or degradation. This is particularly true for items like oils, certain medications, and beverages. Utilizing opaque containers or storing items in dark spaces helps mitigate the negative effects of light exposure.

**Security Measures:** Beyond environmental factors, security is an essential aspect of proper storage. This involves protecting items from theft, damage, or unauthorized access. Implementing secure storage measures not only safeguards the physical integrity of the items but also ensures their intended use.

## Dark Glass Bottles For Preservation

Dark glass bottles play a crucial role in the preservation of light-sensitive substances. The use of dark glass, commonly amber or cobalt blue, is not merely aesthetic but serves a specific purpose in protecting the contents from the harmful effects of light exposure.

**Light Filtering Properties:** The dark color of these glass bottles serves as a natural filter, reducing the transmission of light into the container. This is particularly important for substances like essential oils, medications, and certain beverages that are prone to degradation when exposed to light.

**UV Radiation Protection:** Ultraviolet (UV) radiation, present in natural and artificial light, can accelerate the deterioration of many substances. Dark glass bottles act as a barrier, blocking a significant portion of UV rays and preventing them from reaching and affecting the contents. This is especially critical for preserving the potency of pharmaceuticals and the flavor of light-sensitive beverages.

**Extended Shelf Life:** The use of dark glass bottles can contribute to extending the shelf life of products. By minimizing the impact of light, the degradation processes are slowed down, allowing the contents to remain more stable and effective over an extended period.

**Preservation of Aroma and Flavor:** For products where aroma and flavor are paramount, such as certain oils and spirits, dark glass bottles offer a protective shield against light-induced changes. This is vital for maintaining the intended sensory qualities of the product, ensuring that the end consumer experiences it as intended by the producer.

**Environmental Considerations:** Additionally, the use of dark glass bottles aligns with environmental consciousness. These bottles are often preferred over clear glass or plastic options because they provide protection without the need for additional chemical additives. This not only benefits the stored products but also contributes to sustainable packaging practices.

# Shelf Life And Expiry

Understanding shelf life and expiry is crucial for consumers and producers alike. Shelf life refers to the period during which a product remains suitable for consumption or use, while expiry indicates the point beyond which the product is deemed unsafe or ineffective. This knowledge empowers consumers to make informed choices and helps producers manage inventory effectively.

**Factors Influencing Shelf Life:**

- **Product Composition:** The ingredients and composition of a product play a significant role in determining its shelf life. For example, products with natural ingredients may have a shorter shelf life compared to those with artificial preservatives.

- **Packaging:** The type of packaging used can impact shelf life. Air-tight and light-resistant packaging helps protect products from environmental factors that can accelerate deterioration.

- **Storage Conditions:** As discussed earlier, proper storage techniques are directly linked to shelf life. Products stored in optimal conditions are likely to have a longer shelf life compared to those exposed to unfavorable environments.

- **Preservatives:** The inclusion of preservatives can extend the shelf life of certain products by inhibiting microbial growth and chemical reactions. However, consumer preferences for natural products have led to a shift away from extensive preservative use.

**Understanding Expiry Dates:**

- **Legal Requirements:** In many jurisdictions, including expiration dates on products is a legal requirement. This ensures that consumers have clear information about the timeline for safe consumption or use.

- **Safety Concerns:** Expiry dates are primarily about safety. Beyond this date, the product may pose risks to health due to the potential growth of harmful bacteria, loss of efficacy in medications, or changes in the chemical composition of certain items.

- **Quality vs. Safety:** It's essential for consumers to differentiate between the quality of a product and its safety. While some products may be safe beyond their expiry date, they might not deliver the intended quality. This is particularly true for items like vitamins or certain foods.

- **Responsibility of Producers:** Producers bear the responsibility of conducting thorough testing to determine accurate shelf life and expiry dates. Clear and accurate labeling is crucial for building consumer trust and ensuring safety.

# HERBAL TINCTURES IN DAILY LIFE

*Incorporating Tinctures
into Your Routine*

In the realm of holistic wellness, the incorporation of tinctures into your daily routine has gained significant popularity. Tinctures are liquid extracts, typically made by soaking herbs or other plant materials in alcohol or vinegar. They offer a convenient and potent way to integrate the benefits of herbs into your lifestyle. Let's delve into the various ways you can seamlessly infuse tinctures into your routine.

**1. Start with Understanding Your Needs:**

Before incorporating tinctures, identify your specific wellness goals. Whether it's better sleep, reduced stress, or improved immunity, different herbs cater to distinct needs. Knowing your objectives ensures a targeted approach to integrating tinctures into your daily regimen.

**2. Choose the Right Tincture:**

Tinctures come in a variety of formulations, each with unique properties. For example, lavender tinctures are renowned for their calming effects, while echinacea tinctures are often used to boost immunity. Consider consulting with a herbalist or holistic health practitioner to select the tinctures that align with your goals.

**3. Incorporate into Morning Rituals:**

Morning routines set the tone for the day, and incorporating tinctures can enhance this ritual. **Start your day by adding a few drops of an energizing tincture, such as ginseng or peppermint, to your morning beverage.** This not only imparts a burst of natural energy but also provides a moment of mindfulness as you prepare for the day ahead.

**4. Midday Pick-Me-Up:**

As the day progresses, consider a midday pick-me-up with a tincture that aids focus and concentration. **Rhodiola or ginkgo biloba tinctures can be particularly effective in combating afternoon fatigue and enhancing cognitive function.** A few drops under the tongue can provide a quick and discreet boost without the need for caffeine.

**5. Evening Relaxation Practices:**

Transitioning from the hustle of the day to a calm evening is crucial for overall well-being. Tinctures can play a pivotal role in creating a serene evening routine.

**Morning Rituals**

Morning rituals are the foundation of a productive and balanced day. **Infusing intentionality into your morning routine can set a positive tone and enhance your overall well-being.**

**1. Mindful Mornings:**

Begin your day with mindfulness. **Incorporate practices such as meditation or deep breathing exercises to center yourself.** This mindful start can create a sense of calm that resonates throughout the day.

**2. Hydration Ritual:**

Hydration is key to kickstarting your metabolism and enhancing alertness. **Consider infusing your morning routine with herbal teas or infused water to add flavor and therapeutic benefits.** Ginger and lemon tinctures can be excellent additions for a refreshing twist.

**3. Nutrient-Rich Breakfast:**

Fuel your body with a nutrient-rich breakfast. **Incorporate whole foods, such as fruits, nuts, and seeds, to provide sustained energy.** Consider adding adaptogenic herbs like ashwagandha or holy basil to support your body's resilience to stress.

**4. Technology Detox:**

Resist the urge to check your phone immediately upon waking. **Allow yourself at least 30 minutes of tech-free time in the morning to avoid information overload and set a positive tone for the day.**

**Evening Relaxation Practices**

Creating a calming evening routine is essential for winding down and preparing your body and mind for restful sleep. **Incorporate these practices into your evenings for a serene and rejuvenating end to the day.**

## 1. Digital Detox:

An hour before bedtime, **disconnect from electronic devices. The blue light emitted from screens can interfere with melatonin production, disrupting your sleep-wake cycle.** Instead, engage in relaxing activities such as reading a book or practicing gentle stretches.

## 2. Herbal Infusions:

**Chamomile and valerian root tinctures can be excellent additions to your evening routine.** Prepare a soothing herbal tea or add a few drops of these tinctures to a warm beverage to promote relaxation and prepare your body for sleep.

## 3. Mindful Reflection:

Take a few minutes for mindful reflection before bedtime. **Journaling about your day, expressing gratitude, or practicing mindfulness meditation can help release any lingering stress and promote a restful night's sleep.**

## 4. Create a Comfortable Sleep Environment:

Ensure your bedroom is conducive to sleep. **Dim the lights, keep the room cool, and invest in a comfortable mattress and pillows.** A comfortable sleep environment enhances the quality of your rest.

# CASE STUDIES AND SUCCESS STORIES

*Real-Life Experiences with
Herbal Tinctures*

Herbal tinctures have long been a staple in traditional medicine, and their resurgence in modern times has sparked a wave of interest and experimentation. Many individuals share profound real-life experiences attesting to the benefits of herbal tinctures in managing various health concerns.

## 1. Holistic Approach to Wellness

One of the key aspects of herbal tinctures is their holistic approach to wellness. Unlike some conventional medications that target specific symptoms, herbal tinctures often work synergistically with the body, addressing underlying issues. **This holistic approach is evident in the diversity of herbs used in tinctures, each contributing to overall well-being.** Users often report a sense of balance and harmony in their bodies, transcending the relief of specific symptoms.

## 2. Personalized Healing Journeys

Herbal tinctures provide a platform for personalized healing journeys. Individuals with different health conditions can tailor their usage to meet specific needs. **The adaptability of herbal tinctures allows users to create a unique blend that suits their body's requirements.** This personalization fosters a sense of empowerment and involvement in one's own health, contributing to a more proactive approach to well-being.

## 3. Enhanced Absorption and Quick Action

One striking aspect of real-life experiences with herbal tinctures is the enhanced absorption and rapid onset of action. Unlike some traditional herbal remedies, tinctures are often alcohol-based, facilitating quicker absorption into the bloodstream. **This speed of action is particularly appreciated by individuals seeking prompt relief from symptoms or looking to support their immune system efficiently.** Users often report feeling the effects sooner compared to other forms of herbal supplementation.

## 4. Integrating Tradition with Modern Lifestyles

Herbal tinctures seamlessly blend traditional wisdom with modern lifestyles. Many individuals find solace in the fact that they can incorporate time-tested remedies into their fast-paced lives. **The convenience of tinctures allows for easy integration into daily routines, making herbal remedies more accessible to a wider audience.** This merging of tradition with contemporary living enhances the overall appeal of herbal tinctures.

## Improved Health Conditions

The journey towards improved health conditions is a multifaceted experience, and herbal tinctures play a pivotal role in this transformative process.

## 1. Alleviation of Chronic Conditions

Real-life testimonials often highlight the efficacy of herbal tinctures in alleviating chronic conditions. Whether it's managing pain, reducing inflammation, or addressing autoimmune disorders, individuals report a significant improvement in their health status. **The gradual yet consistent impact on chronic issues showcases the sustained benefits of incorporating herbal tinctures into one's health regimen.**

## 2. Support for Mental Health

In the realm of mental health, herbal tinctures are gaining recognition for their supportive role. **Certain herbs, such as adaptogens, are known for their ability to modulate stress responses and promote mental resilience.** Users share experiences of reduced anxiety, improved sleep, and a general sense of calmness after integrating these tinctures into their daily routine. This holistic approach to mental health resonates with those seeking natural alternatives.

## 3. Boosting Immune Function

Anecdotes abound regarding the immune-boosting properties of herbal tinctures. **Specific herbs, like echinacea and elderberry, are celebrated for their ability to strengthen the immune system.** Users report fewer instances of illness and a quicker recovery when they do fall ill. The preventive aspect of herbal tinctures contributes to an overall improvement in health by reducing the frequency and severity of illnesses.

## 4. Addressing Gut Health

The intricate connection between gut health and overall well-being is a focal point in many health journeys. Herbal tinctures, featuring digestive herbs such as ginger and peppermint, contribute to maintaining a healthy gut. **Improved digestion, reduced bloating, and enhanced nutrient absorption are common themes in user experiences, highlighting the significant impact of herbal tinctures on gut health.**

## Positive Lifestyle Changes

Beyond the realm of physical health, the impact of herbal tinctures extends into fostering positive lifestyle changes. These changes are often interconnected, creating a holistic transformation in individuals' lives.

## 1. Mindful Living Practices

Users frequently express a shift towards mindful living when incorporating herbal tinctures into their routines. **The act of preparing and consuming tinctures becomes a ritual, fostering a sense of mindfulness and presence.** This intentional approach to self-care often extends to other aspects of life, promoting a more conscious and balanced lifestyle.

## 2. Sustainable and Eco-Friendly Choices

The conscious choice of herbal tinctures aligns with a growing awareness of sustainable and eco-friendly living. **Many tinctures are sourced from organic herbs, emphasizing a commitment to environmental well-being.** Users who value sustainability find that their health choices extend beyond personal benefits, contributing to a more significant ecological impact.

## 3. Connection with Nature

Herbal tinctures serve as a conduit for individuals to reconnect with nature in the midst of modern, technology-driven lives. **The cultivation of herbs, the process of making tinctures, and the incorporation of nature-derived remedies bring individuals closer to the natural world.** This reconnection often sparks a renewed appreciation for the healing power of plants and a desire to explore other facets of holistic living.

## 4. Empowerment through Knowledge

A common thread in positive lifestyle changes is the empowerment that comes with knowledge. **Understanding the properties of different herbs, their historical uses, and the science behind herbal tinctures empowers individuals to make informed decisions about their health.** This newfound knowledge often extends beyond herbal remedies, influencing choices in nutrition, exercise, and overall well-being.

# FREQUENTLY ASKED QUESTIONS

## *Addressing Common Concerns*

Addressing common concerns about a product or service is crucial for building trust and ensuring customer satisfaction. One of the primary concerns that customers often have is the safety and reliability of the product. To alleviate these concerns, it's essential to provide transparent information about the product's manufacturing process, quality control measures, and any certifications it may have obtained. Additionally, highlighting customer reviews and testimonials can offer real-life experiences, showcasing the positive impact the product has had on others.

Another common concern revolves around the product's environmental impact. In today's eco-conscious world, customers are increasingly concerned about sustainability. To address this, companies should be transparent about their eco-friendly practices, such as the use of recyclable materials, reduced carbon footprint, and any initiatives they have in place to contribute to environmental conservation.

Furthermore, addressing concerns about the product's longevity and durability is crucial. Provide detailed information about the materials used, testing procedures, and any warranties or guarantees offered. This not only instills confidence in the customer but also sets realistic expectations regarding the product's lifespan.

## Interaction with Medications

Understanding how a product interacts with medications is a critical concern for consumers, particularly when it comes to health and wellness products. To address this concern, it's imperative to provide detailed information about potential interactions and side effects. **Highlighting key points** about the product's compatibility with common medications can assist consumers in making informed decisions.

Moreover, consulting with healthcare professionals before integrating a new product into one's routine is highly advisable. Emphasize the importance of seeking medical advice to ensure that the product aligns with individual health conditions and does not negatively interact with prescribed medications.

Additionally, providing a comprehensive list of ingredients and their potential effects on different medications is essential. This information empowers consumers to make educated choices, promoting responsible usage.

To further address concerns about product safety, companies should conduct thorough clinical trials and share the results transparently. Highlight any certifications or endorsements from healthcare professionals to reinforce the product's reliability.

## Appropriate Usage for Children and Pets

When marketing a product intended for use by children or pets, addressing concerns related to their well-being is paramount. **Enumerating key points** about the appropriate usage of the product for children and pets can serve as a quick reference for concerned consumers.

Start by clearly stating any age or weight restrictions, ensuring that customers are aware of the product's suitability for specific age groups or sizes of pets. Emphasize the importance of following recommended guidelines to prevent any adverse effects.

In the case of products designed for children, providing information on child-safe materials, potential choking hazards, and adherence to safety standards is essential. Clearly communicate any precautions parents should take to ensure a secure environment for their children while using the product.

For products intended for pets, consider including information on the potential impact on their health, proper dosage, and any veterinarian recommendations. This not only demonstrates a commitment to the well-being of animals but also reinforces the product's credibility.

# THE FUTURE OF HERBAL TINCTURES

*Growing Popularity in
Modern Wellness*

In recent years, there has been a notable surge in the popularity of modern wellness practices. This trend is not just a fleeting fad but represents a fundamental shift in the way individuals perceive and prioritize their health. Modern wellness encompasses a holistic approach to well-being, focusing on physical, mental, and emotional health. It goes beyond traditional healthcare and embraces a proactive stance, emphasizing prevention rather than just treatment. As people become more health-conscious, there's a growing interest in activities such as mindfulness, yoga, and personalized nutrition plans.

The allure of modern wellness lies in its ability to cater to the diverse needs of individuals. **Customization** is a key aspect, as wellness programs are often tailored to suit personal preferences, schedules, and health goals.

This adaptability ensures that individuals are more likely to stick to their wellness routines, fostering long-term benefits. The variety of options available, from fitness apps to meditation platforms, caters to different preferences, making wellness practices more accessible to a broader audience.

One driving force behind the popularity of modern wellness is the increasing awareness of the mind-body connection. Many are recognizing that mental well-being is intrinsically linked to physical health. This paradigm shift has led to the integration of practices such as meditation and mindfulness in daily routines. The idea that a healthy mind contributes to overall well-being has spurred interest in practices that promote mental resilience and emotional balance.

Furthermore, social media has played a pivotal role in popularizing modern wellness. Platforms like Instagram and TikTok have become hubs for wellness influencers, sharing their journeys and inspiring others to embark on their paths to well-being. The visual and relatable nature of these platforms creates a sense of community, making wellness feel like a shared journey rather than a solitary pursuit.

**Integration with Mainstream Medicine**

Modern wellness is no longer confined to the realm of alternative or complementary medicine. It has increasingly found its place alongside mainstream medical practices, creating a more comprehensive approach to healthcare. The integration of wellness into mainstream medicine signifies a paradigm shift in how healthcare is approached and delivered.

**Collaboration** between wellness practitioners and traditional healthcare professionals has become more commonplace. This collaboration acknowledges the complementary benefits that each approach brings to the table. For instance, a patient recovering from surgery may find the incorporation of mindfulness techniques beneficial for managing pain and stress, enhancing the overall healing process.

In addition to collaboration, many healthcare institutions are incorporating wellness initiatives into their services. Hospitals and clinics now offer wellness programs that encompass nutritional counseling, stress management, and physical fitness. This integration acknowledges the importance of preventive measures in maintaining health and reducing the burden on the healthcare system.

Patients themselves are becoming more proactive in incorporating wellness practices into their treatment plans. Many are seeking a balance between medical interventions and lifestyle changes to optimize their health outcomes. This shift in attitude reflects a growing understanding that addressing the root causes of health issues often requires a multifaceted approach.


## Ongoing Research and Development

The field of modern wellness is dynamic, with ongoing research and development driving innovation and refinement of existing practices. As scientific understanding deepens, new dimensions of wellness are continually being explored, expanding the horizons of what is possible in promoting holistic health.

**Emerging Technologies** play a significant role in the evolution of modern wellness. From wearable devices that track physical activity and vital signs to apps that monitor mental well-being, technology is providing individuals with real-time data and insights into their health. This data-driven approach empowers individuals to make informed decisions about their wellness routines, enhancing the efficacy of their efforts.

The scientific community's interest in the gut-brain axis and the microbiome has opened up new avenues for wellness research. Understanding the intricate relationship between gut health and overall well-being has led to the development of personalized nutrition plans and probiotic interventions. This represents a shift towards more targeted and individualized approaches to wellness, acknowledging that one size does not fit all.

Moreover, ongoing research is debunking myths and validating the efficacy of certain wellness practices. For instance, studies on the benefits of meditation and mindfulness in reducing stress and improving mental health have contributed to the mainstream acceptance of these practices. This integration of evidence-based approaches further solidifies the credibility of modern wellness in the eyes of both the public and healthcare professionals.

# CONCLUSION

## *Recap of Key Takeaways*

In our journey through this insightful exploration, let's reflect on the key takeaways that have illuminated our understanding. The essence of recapping lies in distilling complex information into concise, memorable points.

**1. Knowledge Retention:**

- Understanding the importance of effective learning mechanisms is crucial.
- Utilizing various senses and learning styles enhances information retention.

The human brain thrives on repetition and multi-sensory engagement. This is a fundamental concept in education and cognitive science. The more we revisit and reinforce information, the more likely it is to be retained. Pairing visual aids with verbal explanations, for example, can significantly enhance comprehension.

**2. Application in Real Life:**

- Practical application solidifies theoretical knowledge.
- Bridging the gap between learning and doing is imperative.

Learning gains true value when it can be applied to real-life situations. Knowledge is not merely about accumulating facts; it's about empowering individuals to navigate and contribute to their environment. Encouraging practical exercises and scenarios enhances the transition from theory to practice.

## 3. Continuous Learning:

- Embracing a lifelong learning mindset is essential.
- The world is dynamic; knowledge should evolve accordingly.

The pace of change in today's world demands continuous learning. Embracing the idea that education is not confined to a specific period but is a lifelong journey empowers individuals to adapt to new challenges. It fosters resilience, agility, and a proactive approach to personal and professional growth.

## Encouragement for Readers to Explore the World of Herbal Tinctures

Embarking on the exploration of herbal tinctures opens a world of natural remedies and holistic well-being. The allure lies not only in the diverse plant-based concoctions but also in the centuries-old wisdom that accompanies them.

## 1. Rich Heritage of Herbal Wisdom:

- Herbal remedies have been integral to various cultures throughout history.
- Exploring traditional practices provides insights into the holistic approach to health.

Delving into the world of herbal tinctures is like stepping

into a repository of ancestral knowledge. Different cultures have their unique herbal traditions, each with its distinct set of plants and methods. Understanding these traditions not only enriches one's knowledge but also fosters a deep appreciation for the interconnectedness of nature and well-being.

## 2. Personalized Wellness Journey:

- Herbal tinctures offer a personalized approach to health.
- Tailoring remedies to individual needs is a cornerstone of herbal medicine.

Unlike one-size-fits-all pharmaceuticals, herbal tinctures allow for a customized approach to wellness. The diverse array of herbs and their unique properties enables individuals to address specific health concerns or simply enhance overall well-being. This personalized aspect aligns with the growing trend of holistic and patient-centric healthcare.

## 3. Sustainable and Natural Solutions:

- Herbal tinctures contribute to sustainable and eco-friendly health practices.
- Exploring natural remedies aligns with a global shift towards sustainability.

As environmental consciousness becomes integral to lifestyle choices, herbal tinctures offer a sustainable alternative. Harvesting plants for medicinal purposes, when done responsibly, can be less taxing on the environment compared to the production of synthetic pharmaceuticals. This aligns with the global movement towards embracing natural, eco-friendly solutions.

## 4. Holistic Approach to Healing:

- Herbal tinctures emphasize the interconnectedness of mind, body, and spirit.
- Adopting a holistic approach fosters comprehensive well-being.

Herbal medicine operates on the principle that health is not just the absence of disease but a state of balance and harmony within the body. By addressing the root causes of ailments and considering the interconnectedness of various bodily systems, herbal tinctures offer a holistic approach to healing. This aligns with a broader cultural shift towards holistic well-being.